SO YOU WANT TO BE A THERAPIST?

How to become a Physical or Occupational Therapist

KIRK PAINTER, PT, DPT, CERT. MDT

Doctor of Physical Therapy

ISBN-13: 978-1494995270

Printed in the United States

Because many more applicants apply to physical and occupational therapy schools than are accepted, you should pursue this endeavor very seriously and with fervent effort. Despite the odds, becoming a therapist is well worth the work involved to achieve this goal. With this book, I will outline the steps and tips necessary to place you in the best light possible for the interview and acceptance into one of the many therapy programs. Many of these recommendations are also applicable to physical therapy assistants and occupational therapy assistants (See Chapter 4).

Dedicated to all those who seek to help others by giving of themselves.

CONTENTS

Click on chapters below to jump ahead, then go back
to TOC at top of reader to return to this page.

About the Author

Kirk Painter has been a practicing physical therapist (P.T.) since 1995. He is a credentialed clinical instructor, is certified as a Graston® provider, and is a Certified McKenzie provider. He has served, and continues to serve, as an adjunct faculty at Texas State University. He has also just recently graduated with his doctorate of physical therapy from The University Of Texas Health Science Center, in San Antonio. He is also part owner of two thriving outpatient clinics with diverse clients and services.

Kirk has participated, as an interviewer, for many years in Texas State University interviews with their P.T. school applicants. Since 1995, he has also worked with innumerable employees and volunteers, who have eventually become practicing physical therapists. Through this process of observing, studying, interviewing, and following hundreds of potential students, he has better understood the traits of those who got accepted into school and those who did not make the cut.

He has always harbored a curiosity for science and mechanics. As an eight-year-old, he acquired and then assembled a model human skull that raised a few suspicious eyebrows in his family. He began his college career as a business major, but on a whim happened to try an anatomy class. This class sparked such a curiosity in him that he knew that a degree in business was no longer an option. To confirm his new educational path, he took more biology classes. He also enrolled in an EMT (Emergency Medical Technician) course, while in his first year of college, to further explore his curiosity in the medical field. Since he grew up with horses and cattle, he ultimately pursued an animal science degree. After graduating with a degree in animal science, he worked for the USDA, but kept exploring the medical field possibilities. He finally found physical therapy and knew it was the perfect fit. In 1991, Kirk then took a leap of faith, and went back to school to pursue his new passion. With superb grades, diverse physical therapy volunteer experiences, and a successful interview, he successfully completed P.T. school at Southwest Texas State University (now Texas State University) in 1994.

He has worked at the Physical Therapy & Rehab Concepts San Marcos office since 1995 and has been co-owner and director since 1998.

He is the father of three awesome teenagers, at the time of writing this book, and stays very busy with them, his wife, his business, and school.

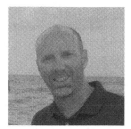

INTRODUCTION

Happiness in your career

If you are reading this, then chances are that either you or someone you care about is interested in a career in physical or occupational therapy. These are truly amazing medical fields with great opportunities and compensation. If you are bright, energetic, passionate about helping people, intrigued by the human body, and enjoy exercise, then this field may be perfect for you! Much of the information and advice in this book is common sense and may sound like general knowledge, however knowing what is required and acting on it, will help put you in the best position of gaining acceptance into one of the many excellent programs offered. I recommend observing therapists in your area to see if what they do is exciting to you. Observe various settings, since there are many, and then decide to pursue this career further if it excites you.

Physical Therapists

What is a physical therapist and what do they do? The 2012 Handbook of Bureau of Labor Statistics states:

"Physical therapists, sometimes referred to as simply PTs, are healthcare professionals who diagnose and treat individuals of all ages, from newborns to the very oldest, who have medical problems or other health-related conditions, illnesses, or injuries that limit their abilities to move and perform functional activities as well as they would like in their daily lives. Physical therapists examine each individual and develop a plan using treatment techniques to promote the ability to move, reduce pain, restore function, and prevent disability. In addition, PTs work with individuals to prevent the loss of mobility before it occurs by developing fitness and wellness-oriented programs for healthier and more active lifestyles."

Physical therapists typically need a doctoral degree in physical therapy. All states require physical therapists to be licensed.

According to the Bureau of Labor Statistics, the average annual salary for physical therapists was $79,860 in May 2012 and the job growth is expected to increase by 36% by the year 2022. For an occupational therapist, it is $75,400 and the increase in job growth is expected to be 29% over the same period. Physical and occupational therapists are ranked very highly in the top jobs in the nation. The want-ads frequently list therapy openings and include hefty sign-on bonuses. I know, as a physical therapist, I receive offers via phone calls and emails frequently. The recruiters that call me will ask if I know any therapists looking for work, since I am not looking for another position. This clearly demonstrates that there are more positions than applicants. Good salaries, plenty of job opportunities, and satisfying work make physical or occupational therapy an amazing career, but the best part is the differences you make in people's lives. Helping others is very satisfying, and at the end of the day you know you have made a difference.

Occupational Therapist

The 2012 Handbook of Bureau of Labor Statistics states: Occupational therapists (O.T.s) typically do the following:

- "Observe patients doing tasks, ask the patient questions, and review the patient's medical history.
- Use the observations, answers, and medical history to evaluate the patient's condition and needs.
- Establish a treatment plan for patients, laying out the types of activities and specific goals to be accomplished.
- Help people with various disabilities with different tasks, such as helping an older person with poor memory use a computer, or leading an autistic child in play activities.
- Demonstrate exercises that can help relieve pain for people with chronic conditions, such as joint stretches for arthritis sufferers.
- Evaluate a patient's home or workplace and identify how it can be better suited to the patient's health needs.
- Educate a patient's family and employer about how to accommodate and care for the patient. Recommend special equipment, such as wheelchairs and eating aids, and instruct patients how to use that equipment.
- Assess and record patients' activities and progress for evaluating clients, for billing, and for reporting to physicians and other healthcare providers."

Occupational therapists need a master's or doctorate degree from an accredited occupational therapy program. Occupational therapists, like physical therapists, must also be licensed.

It is worth it

To summarize, not only is the salary great, but the satisfaction is extremely high as well! As a practicing therapist, I can say that I still enjoy working each day. In fact, I find I am enjoying it more and more every year. In my outpatient practice, I see many return patients from years past. This scenario is similar to old friends dropping by, always picking up right where we left off – familiar, comfortable, and friendly. Although it can be demanding, being a therapist is truly very satisfying. In my practice, each therapist spends several hours each week with his/her patients. You will get to know your patients and subsequently develop a bond with them. As the therapist, you are entrusted to help the patient and they, in turn, have to trust that you will help them. The common desire that both the patient and the therapist have is to improve patient wellness. This goal helps form the bond between clinician and patient, and that common goal is the part that makes the job satisfying. You each learn about the other's career, political views, family, and hobbies. Almost every patient I see is interesting, nice and fun, regardless of age. Your patients will vary widely in their own expectations and personalities; you have to be flexible and adapt to each person's differences to be effective in this or any public service field.

Within this book are numerous links to websites. It is possible that with time, these links may no longer function. However, the name of the site is listed, so you will still be able to research if the links somehow fail. I recommend re-reading this book or various sections multiple times to help commit some important actions to memory.

Chapter 1

Personality

Do you have one that will fit?

Personality traits

To be successful in this field, you need to be patient, empathetic, open-minded, and detail-oriented. You need to be able to creatively problem-solve, and most of all, be able to invest all you can to help your patient - using all your energy and skills. A good therapist has the ability to motivate a person who is anxious and in pain. The patient has to trust and believe that the therapist can facilitate a return to normalcy. As a therapist, you must learn and master patience while also adapting to the many patient personality types. Most of the patients you encounter are in pain and stressed due to their new-found disability. You need to be cognizant of this when interacting with them, understanding that some patients are very apprehensive, scared, doubtful, or just irritated with the entire medical process. You need to have the skills to allay any fears or doubts so that you and the patient can work together as a trusting team. Being detail-oriented, showing leadership and authority are very important to be successful, not only as a physical therapist, but as a leader in the field. Creative problem solving is required daily because not everyone or every diagnosis or problem will fit into a neat little box. By applying what you have learned in P.T. or O.T. school and coupling this with your clinical experiences, you are often the one who finds alternate ways to address problems that the patient or doctor may not have thought of yet.

I have interviewed countless P.T. applicants at Texas State University and have seen even more volunteers, interns, and technicians who were all aspiring to become therapists. After more than 20 years of observing, watching, interviewing, challenging, and studying these individuals, I have observed the actions and behaviors that are required to gain admission into school. A professor I know says that interns, volunteers, or students "either get it or they don't." This phrase is so simple, but absolutely true. To *get it* you have to be: bright, energetic, open-minded, humble, a quick learner, and be able to understand and relate well with people. Bright: Have a good memory and be able to understand concepts easily. Energetic: Be mentally engaged and aware of <u>all</u> needs around you, efficient, and always ready to help. Open minded: Be accepting of new ideas and ready and willing to perform tasks with which you are unaware. Humble: This trait is very important! Even if you have all the successful traits needed, if you are brash and exude superiority, then you will fail in your attempt to become a therapist.

Note: You should be confident, but not over confident.

A quick learner: Be fast to grasp new instructions needing to be shown or told something just once. Be relatable: You will need to "read people." You need to speak his or her language. People usually like to talk about themselves and if you ask questions about them, you will learn a great deal about life and careers. For example, if you have someone's great-grandmother, who worked several jobs her entire life, relate with her on her work ethic and her family. If you have an older ranch hand, then talk to him or her about the ranch life. These individuals will open up and see you as a great conversationalist. Of course, you need to possess a natural curiosity about these individuals, which can help you understand what he or she wants to get out of therapy. These patients may have goals such as: getting up on a horse or lifting a 20-pound great-grandchild. If the therapist is unaware of these goals, tell him or her about what you have talked about. Experienced therapists can tell in a very short time which volunteer, intern, or aide will be quick to grasp the complexities of both patient care and customer service. Regarding customer service, an orthopedic surgeon I know states that "a mediocre doctor who has a great bedside manner will do well with fans as patients." He affirmed what I have told countless P.T. students during their clinical rotations at our clinic. You need to keep the patients' overall well-being foremost in your thoughts while treating them. The therapist's sense of who will be a successful applicant is supported by recalling the traits of those who ultimately do succeed. Many practicing therapists appraise these aspiring students without really thinking about it directly. Whether thinking about it directly or not, therapists can recall who ultimately succeeds and who does not. We develop a sense of what it takes to succeed in this field and what encompasses all that can prevent one from getting invited to an interview. The qualities of the applicant are very important, we look at the traits a person possesses, and his/her work ethic as well. To sum this up, be a genuine, happy, smart, cheerful giver – all of the time. This equates to you being eager to make a difference in the facility and with the patients no matter how trivial your tasks may seem to you.

Hint: If you are fortunate enough to work with other technicians or interns, observe who is very good at their job. Make sure that your assessment of the successful individual(s) is correct in that the therapists, staff, and patients all respect the aide or technician and count on them for successful day-to-day work. Once you identify them, study his or her personal interactions and work ethic, and then try to emulate the best parts of these behaviors.

The government's Bureau of Labor and Statistics website (**http://www.bls.gov/ooh/Healthcare/Physical-therapists.htm**) lists information that generalizes some important qualities of a P.T.

Important Qualities of a P.T.

Compassion. *Physical therapists are often drawn to the profession in part by a desire to help people. They work with people who are in pain and must have empathy to help their patients.*

Detail oriented. *Like other healthcare providers, physical therapists should have strong analytical and observational skills to diagnose a patient's problem, evaluate treatments, and provide safe, effective care.*

Dexterity. *Physical therapists should be comfortable using their hands to provide manual therapy and therapeutic exercises.*

Interpersonal skills. *Because physical therapists spend their time interacting with patients, they should enjoy working with people. They must be able to explain treatment programs, educate their patients, and listen to the patients' concerns to provide effective therapy.*

Physical stamina. *Physical therapists spend much of their time on their feet, moving as they work with their patients. They should enjoy physical activity.*

Important Qualities of an O.T.

http://www.bls.gov/ooh/Healthcare/Occupational-therapists.htm

Communication skills*. Occupational therapists have to be able to explain clearly what they want their patients to do.*

Compassion*. Occupational therapists are usually drawn to the profession by a desire to help people and improve the daily lives of others.*

Interpersonal skills*. Because occupational therapists spend their time teaching and explaining therapies to patients, they should inspire trust and respect from their clients.*

Listening skills*. Occupational therapists must be able to listen attentively to what their patients tell them.*

Patience*. Dealing with injuries, illnesses, and disabilities is frustrating for many people. Occupational therapists should be patient in order to provide quality care for the people they serve.*

Writing skills*. Occupational therapists must be able to explain clearly to others on the patient's medical team what they are doing and how it is going.*

Ch. 1 Summary:

- You need to be patient, empathetic, flexible, and detail oriented.
- Invest your time and energy in the patients' well-being.
- You need to have the skills to allay any fears or doubts so that you and the patient work together as a trusting team.
- To *have the right stuff* you have to be: bright, energetic, open minded, humble, a quick learner, and be able to understand people, relating to them well.
- You have to be an effective oral and written communicator.
- You need to understand non-verbal communication of someone who is in pain and/or anxious.

Chapter 2

Preparation

Before embarking into a rigorous and competitive, albeit rewarding, career like physical or occupational therapy, you need to be 100% certain that it is for you. Step one: The best way to know if it is the right choice is to learn all you can about this field. Besides internet research, I strongly advise that you observe at multiple clinical settings to see if you like it or not. Talk to the therapists, the aides, and the volunteers to get insight regarding these exciting fields. Learn as much as you can based on this real life experience of witnessing what really happens in a clinical setting. If you leave excited about it after your first day of exposure, then you are on your way, and the future time and effort needed to succeed will be easier. Step two: can you make the grades? The average overall GPA for accepted (PTCAS) applicants in 2009-2010 was 3.47 out of 4.0. The 2012-2013 accepted GPA was 3.54 out of 4.0, and is trending upwards yearly. In case you have never calculated college grades, let me put it in perspective. Let's look at two 16-hour semesters. With the first semester, you make all A's and one B (in one three-hour course). This would average to a 3.75 GPA semester for you. Then the next semester you make all A's except for two B's in a four-hour and a three-hour course, respectfully. This would be a 3.56 semester for you. Average the 3.75 and 3.56 which equals one year with a 3.65 GPA. Understand that if you make a 3.5 GPA overall, you are only getting close to the average admittance score of *3.54,* as discussed above. Why be average and not give yourself an edge by doing better? Strive for perfection and your odds of getting into school improve drastically. This is where your ability to endure delayed gratification is very important. I had an obvious thought process about my courses in P.T. school. I thought, "I need to do the best I can, making the best grades possible so I have the answers needed to help my future patients." This thought process was the same when I became an EMT. While keeping your eye on superb grades and a GRE (http://www.takethegre.com/) score (if applicable for your chosen school), you should then check into the schools you wish to apply to and make sure you have all the prerequisites and grades needed.

> Note: Each school is a little different in its requirements for entry, and you should pick the school that fits you best.

You need to prove to these schools, and yourself, that you are sure of your choice. You should show them you are serious and informed by volunteering or working at multiple locations such as your local hospital, rehab facility, home health, and outpatient clinics. Most schools will not be impressed if you only have experience in one type of setting. You may even try participating in activities such as the Special Olympics or with Hippotherapy (where horses are used as the medium of treatment). You should also study the current national and state level political trends through the APTA or AOTA websites. You will also find topics of interest directly related to our field at the state level. Your state will have its own association; Texas has the TPTA. Do not underestimate the information at national, state, and local levels.

You need to really prove your understanding about current trends, or the interviewing faculty will know you just skimmed the information to pacify them during the interview. I have been asked poorly-researched questions that I know the applicant was asking just so he/she could *try* to impress me with his/her "knowledge." However, it was instantly apparent that the potential applicant did not fully read or try to actually understand the topic. Do your homework and invest your time and energy so that you impress those who can help you get into this amazing career.

What faculty says:

I interviewed P.T. and O.T. school professors and chairs of departments to obtain their valuable insight. I asked common questions that many aspiring therapy school applicants have asked me and other therapists. The following questions are general and are focused on facilitating entrance into a professional graduate program.

Question One:

What are the top three to five things that a candidate needs to have to facilitate their acceptance into P.T. school?

Dr. Barbara Sanders, PT, PhD, SCS - Department Chair of the Texas State Physical Therapy Program answered below:

- She stated: "*1. Good grades. 2. Good GRE scores. 3. Knowledge about the profession. 4. Knowledge about the academic program. 5. Good people skills.*"

Catherine Ortega, Ed.D, PT, ATC, OCS. Associate Professor,

Chairperson at UTSCSA answered the same question via an email. Her response to the same question was paraphrased below:

- *Keep up GPA -- retake classes with a C because the cut-off point in science is a 3.0/4.0. Really take your time with the personal statement. This statement is the only view that we get of the person on paper. To write 'I want to help people," or "I think the human body is fascinating" is not really a good answer. Everyone says that. We are looking for something that distinguishes the applicant, about their reasons to be a PT.* She summarized that they should know about the profession. *She stated, "to be sure that they should participate in service activities outside of school and also be a leader in service activities. EVERYONE does service, we are looking for leaders in service. Be sure to ask someone to write a GOOD Letter of Recommendation. If it says just 'shows up on time', 'is presentable', it not really a helpful letter of recommendation."* How is the communication? Interpersonal skills, do they ask good questions? Etc. We do not deduct for a 'mediocre or poor' letter, but it just does not add anything to an application.

Dr. Steve Spivey, P.T., DPT, Clinical Assistant Professor and the Director of Clinical Education at Texas State University answered below:

- *"Grades, good references, variety of work experience, strong interview skills, well written essays."*

Susan P. Denham, Ed.D, MS, OTR/L, CHT, Department Chair/Professor of Occupational Therapy at Alabama State University. She answered the same question, but regarding O.T. students:

- *"GPA- Overall GPA and Prerequisite GPA are very important"*
- *"Well written (no mistakes) essay. Good interview and personal skills – a sense of maturity and knowledge of the school and profession. Call, email, or come to open houses at the school to assure you are meeting all the requirements."*

Question Two:

What do you feel are the best traits to possess as a successful applicant?

- Dr. Sanders responded with: *"Maturity, communication of critical thinking and problem solving skills."*
- Dr. Ortega responded with: *"[I feel it is] a strong application on paper AND a good understanding of the profession."* She suggested the applicants *cruise the APTA and TPTA websites so that they know what the issues are. "PREPARE for the interview. Don't just give a 'stock' regular answer to questions. Make sure to ask some thoughtful questions that show you looked up the program or the faculty. PRACTICE answering questions, this will definitely help you."*
- Dr. Spivey states: *"Being comfortable in their own skin, professionalism, maturity and passion for P.T."*
- Dr. Denham states that the applicants need to be: *Creative, well spoken, [show] curiosity and [have a] good work ethic.*

Question Three:

How heavily do schools look at the applicant's extracurricular activities/clubs/sports, and does it help get them noticed?

- Dr. Sanders stated: *"It is an area that is included in our review of the holistic view of the applicant – can the individual balance a number of commitments – school, work, athletic participation, service in the community, family, etc."*
- Dr. Spivey stated: *"Not heavily, a good starting point for the interview."*
- Dr. Denham states: *"Only if the activities link to the profession - for example: working at a special-need's camp, or to a VERY small degree if it relates to a slightly lower GPA, for example a Basketball player who has a 3.2 GPA."*

Question Four:

What are the common mistakes that applicants make?

- Dr. Sanders stated: *"They do not follow directions. They do not do their homework."* The homework she speaks about includes knowing the school, the steps in the application process, and the professors.
- Dr. Ortega reported: *Poor letters of recommendation, and mediocre 'pat' answers to the personal statement. They do not give enough information when questioned, or worse, they talk too long once the question is answered. They miss the deadlines. The applicant fails to ensure all necessary steps are followed in the process. If a document is missing*

such as a letter of recommendation or transcript, the folder never gets seen.

- Dr. Denham stated: *By far, the biggest mistake is NOT FOLLOWING DIRECTIONS! They should be aware of all requirements, view the website, meet deadlines etc.*
- *Another mistake is taking the advice of an advisor (at their current school) and not checking with us. For example: "My advisor said Biology could be used for Anatomy."*

Note: No mistakes is key. Check and re-check. Know your dates and deadlines.

Now from a successful applicant in the Texas State program.

I also asked *Jeffrey Bierman, a* current student in P.T. school, a few common questions:

What are the top three to five things you did to gain admission into P.T. school?

- *"My hours of volunteer work/observation in different settings. I had 244 hours of volunteer work/observation. When completing those hours, I observed pediatric, orthopedic, neurologic, lymphedema, acute care, and wound therapy. I feel this gave me a great advantage over the other applicants.*
- *My persistence. It took me three attempts to make it into physical therapy school. Each time I applied, I made it further into the process. My first year (I was still in undergrad), I did not receive an interview. On my second try, I received an interview, made alternate, but did not*

become accepted. On my third try, I ma[...]
then received the call that I was accepted.[...]
interviewers saw that I did not become unmo[...]
my goal of becoming a PT by being denied for t[...]

- *My personality. My second attempt at PT school, t[...]*
a snow storm the day before my interview, and the
University closed campus. Because of this, the program
decided to do phone interviews. I became an end of the lis[...]
alternate. I feel that my personality did not come through
during the phone interview which hurt my chances. The
next year, I had the one-on-one interviews and made 2nd
alternate which led to me becoming accepted."

What do you feel are the best traits to possess as a successful applicant?

- *"I believe the best trait you can have is to show that you*
care. Physical Therapy is a career where you are put in a
position to help people get their lives back. You've got to
show that in your interview to even have a chance. A
physical therapy program doesn't want to put out someone
who doesn't care. Another trait is that you are motivated. A
PT program wants to know that you are willing to push
through the rough times during PT school."

Do or did your extracurricular activities/clubs help get you noticed?

- *"I think extracurricular activities helped the process.*
Physical therapists have to interact with a whole lot of

He makes great points and each one should be taken to heart and applied. I recommend speaking to as many accepted P.T. students as possible and asking what he or she think helped him or her get into P.T. school. If you have low grades in some courses, I recommend you re-take those courses and make better grades which will accomplish two things: 1. You will impress the faculty reviewing your file by showing them your dedication. 2. You will increase your GPA which increases odds of being accepted.

I also asked *Nicole Indrieri,* a recent P.T. graduate from The University of Texas Health Science Center at San Antonio, the same questions:

What are the top three to five things you did that you feel got you into P.T. school?

- *"Persistence.*

- *Volunteering in a variety of PT settings (NICU, outpatient, inpatient, SNF, school).*
- *Demonstrated good work ethic, eagerness to learn, and volunteered for approximately 2 months at each location to develop a relationship with potential references.*
- *Researching current events in PT, knowing the professors and general stats at each school before the interviews.*
- *Met with head of PT department before applying!*
- *My work history on my resume was also important during the interview process - especially the decision to change careers."*

What do you feel are the best traits to possess as a successful applicant?

- *"Confidence, positive attitude.*
- *Eagerness to learn, and willingness to make mistakes during the process.*
- *Good grades in undergrad!*
- *Persistence!"*

Do or did your extracurricular activities/clubs help get you noticed?

- *"I think so ... It gave us something to talk about during the interview process and demonstrated commitment."*

My own view on why you have to work hard and stand out.

I recall that after I was admitted, I learned that out of more than 600 applicants, about 50% were excluded based on incomplete paperwork or incomplete requirements. Out of those remaining ±

300 applicants, about 120 were invited to be interviewed. Out of the 120, about 25% were accepted, which turned out to be my class of 32 students. This ratio of one successful entry to every 17-19 applications remains relatively true even today. This demonstrates how hard you have to work to eventually be accepted into a professional school. You can do it, but you have to work very hard to make great grades, get experience, and study the profession. You should be prepared to apply to multiple schools, and possibly re-apply the following year(s).

Ch. 2 Summary:

- It is very important to begin this entire preparatory process as soon as possible. I recommend starting in high school or in your freshman year in college. The more diverse your work or volunteer experiences, the better.
- Quickly ascertain if this field fits you by observing it first-hand.
  - Note that there are many types of facilities that do different types of therapy; don't make a decision based on one visit in just one type of setting.
- Make competitive grades – 3.5 GPA or greater, if possible.
- Know the schools and faculty.
- Follow the steps required and complete the application process accurately and within the stated time frame.
- Use the school's check-off sheets if they have them or make your own so you can track your steps and progress.

Chapter 3

Schools

Physical Therapy

Most schools will now require an undergraduate degree first. Pick a degree plan that you will enjoy and one that can help you find a good job if you don't get into P.T. or O.T. school. Many students choose an exercise and sports science major, but many just choose a science degree that interests them. Talk to your counselors and pick a multi-purpose undergraduate degree. However, also consider picking a degree that allows you to get most, if not all, of the prerequisite classes possible for the therapy schools you choose. Some common core classes needed are: Physics, Chemistry, Anatomy, Physiology, Statistics, Medical Terminology and more. You should check with each school for the requirements. Before starting, you need to know that the costs of P.T. school tuition may range from $12,000 to $40,000 per year.

Numbers

As of June 2012, the Commission on Accreditation in Physical Therapy Education (CAPTE) lists 211 accredited physical therapy schools in the U.S. Some states such as New Mexico, Delaware and Idaho have only one school, while the state of New York has twenty-one programs/schools. All but five schools listed culminate in a doctoral degree. There are 24,848 students enrolled as of 2011-2012. There are 283 accredited physical therapy assistant programs with 10,598 students as of 2011-2012. That makes 35,446 total student slots with about 15-20 applicants per spot, which means there are about 532,000 to 709,000 applicants each year, just through the CAPTE site. By going to **http://www.capteonline.org** you can find a school near you. Using their site, you can also filter the program you want by criteria such as: multiple admission dates, credit for military experience, distance learning, whether it culminates in a master's or doctorate degree, volunteer hours needed, and more. There is also great information about the application requirements for schools listed on the **PTCAS site** at (**http://www.ptcas.org/home.aspx**). The Physical Therapist Centralized Application Service (PTCAS) is a service of the American Physical Therapy Association (APTA) at (**http://apta.org/**). PTCAS allows applicants to use a single application and one set of materials to apply to multiple PT programs. Some states have their own version and are not in the PTCAS directory. Pay close attention to the PTCAS deadlines, which may be different for the school you are applying to. In Texas, we have ApplyTexas at **http://www.applytexas.org**. Some other states may have no centralized options. As stated earlier, an undergraduate degree is usually needed first before considering a program. In general, most schools will require a GPA (grade point average) higher than a 3.0 out of 4.0 and a GRE (The *GRE®* revised General Test) score of at least 1000 (if taken before August 1st, 2011). After August 2011 the minimum GRE scoring to be considered varies, but scaled scores of: 150 in Quantitative reasoning, 150 in Verbal reasoning and a 4.0 for Analytical writing are very competitive. The GRE is typically required to enter graduate school, so check with each school to see if it is indeed required.

> Note: You will need to check the schools to see their exact minimum requirements. I personally consider a 3.5 GPA as a starting point to give you a fighting chance for most programs. Applicants can get in with lower GPA's, but you have a much better chance if you have a 3.5 or higher GPA.

Occupational Therapy

Most O.T. schools now are at the master's level, and require an undergraduate degree before you can apply. Pick a degree plan that you will enjoy and one that can get you a good job if you don't get into O.T. school. Many of the schools take 30-50 students each cycle and it is getting more competitive each year. There may be 300 or more applicants applying for these 30-50 slots, so you need to have good grades, great references, and great experiences. Many of the GPA requirements vary, but range from a 2.8 to 3.0 or even higher. The average GPA of a sitting class in most programs will be around a 3.5 overall, and the cost is about the same as P.T. school.

At the time of writing, there are five accredited schools that offer a doctorate program:

Missouri - Washington University

Nebraska - Creighton University

Ohio – University of Toledo

Pennsylvania – University of the Sciences

Tennessee – Belmont University

The BLS site states, "In March 2013, there were 149 occupational therapy programs accredited by the Accreditation Council for Occupational Therapy Education, part of the American Occupational Therapy Association. . ." There are even more occupational assistant programs offered in most states.

Go to: **http://www.aota.org** and look under _Education and Careers_, and then _Find a school_. You can also try: **http://www.gradschools.com** as well.

To find schools that use the centralized application process, go to: **https://portal**.otcas**.org** and then on the left side of their site click on **Participating Programs** link under their Help section.

Note: Regarding employment or abilities for physical and occupational therapists, there is little to no distinction between having a doctorate, masters, or baccalaureate degree. Over the past decade, there is a trend where more and more programs are advancing to master's or doctorate levels, but employers are still hiring, at all levels, regardless of this educational difference.

Pick your schools

By your sophomore year in college, you should research 8-10 possible schools, note what prerequisite courses they require and then take those classes. Once you have the list of schools you are interested in, go to each school's site and download the reference forms, the requirements forms, and any other information you will need. This information will assist you in the decision process. You will need to know when the applications are due, what the graduation dates are, and have all classes completed prior to the graduate school's deadlines. There are numerous ways to organize each school's information. I recommend using any or all of the following methods:

- You can make a folder in your internet browser or on your desktop with the title of "Schools" then a sub-folder of each school's name under that.
- Within each of the 8-10 school folders, I would save the respective link addresses for the information needed for future reference. Examples:
  - Advising appointments
  - Prerequisites
  - Graduate college requirements
  - Application instructions
  - Contact information
  - Deadline dates
- You can also make physical or digital note cards with each school's information on it (see example in this chapter on pg. 26) and keep that in a digital and/or physical folder for quick reference.

To increase your chances of getting into school, I suggest applying to at least five of the schools you selected. The numbers are on your side; the more schools you apply to, the better the chances are that you may be accepted. Compile the list of potential schools based on location, costs, support systems, and overall fit for you. Based on your research of your five chosen schools, try to match your strengths, the school's location, and your personality with the institution's criteria for entrance. Keep this list of schools because you may have to re-apply next year. It is possible that you may not get an interview to *any* of the schools, and will have to choose which ones to apply to next year/cycle. Hopefully, you will be asked to interview at more than one school, so take that into account regarding potential schedule conflicts, travel time, and preparation time for each school's application process. Study those schools carefully and find out all you can about them including the faculty and the area. When speaking to the faculty, you may ask if there are a few students you could contact. Try to get a few names of some of the graduates or current students and contact them to get their honest opinion about their school. These current or past students can provide insight you will not find in brochures or from the faculty. However, I caution making a decision based on one person's opinion alone; try to get a few opinions. You will want to know why they chose the school, what potential barriers there are, and what is the school *looking for* in an applicant. Everyone is impressed by a knowledgeable applicant, whether it's for a job or for a professional school. You should know when the application deadline is, when the program starts, when the breaks are, when and where the internships are, and lastly when you would graduate. You need to know the professors' backgrounds and specialties – which may match up to your future goals and provide a common ground for conversation – perhaps even in the interview. Know what is unique about each university and why it is a good fit for you. Some schools have a strong manual therapy slant, others may have a more pediatric, sports, or even an amputee/prosthetic focused program. You should be able to confidently answer the interview question: "Why did you choose our school?" or "How do you see yourself fitting into our program and why?" Just be honest. The interviewers can tell if you are just saying what you think they want to hear. If you can get to know any of the therapy school faculty and in-turn if they can get to know you, then you will be at the forefront of their minds in many instances. This interaction increases your chances of getting accepted. You can foster these relations by volunteering in the school's treatment clinic, if they have one. If the therapy school does not have a working clinic, you will have to be known by the faculty from advising appointment(s), or by other courses you may have taken from these individuals.

School locations

Research the cost of living, tuition, fees, grants available, family support nearby, and the job market based on your particular skills. With the rigorous course selection, maintaining even a 15-hour per week job would be very challenging. However, if you have a highly reimbursable skill-set, you may be able to work ten to fifteen hours per week to offset expenses. Most schools will discourage any outside work while in O.T. or P.T. school. You will have to balance your studies and your social life, so don't forget to consider the location regarding your hobbies too. By knowing: the cost of housing and how close it is to the school, the terrain, and the environment, you can see how this may match your hobbies, budget, and holistic needs. I recommend nurturing your hobby(s) which will help you cope with the stress of a professional graduate school, so keep up with it. If you are moving to a distant school, **Payscale.com** has a cost of living comparison calculator that is a perfect tool to compare costs from one city to another. You should also research cost of living index (COLI) and the **ACCRA cost of living index** for more information. Many applicants are married or have a significant other, so you need to consider how easily he/she can find work, noting if the area will support his/her skills and subsequently, you.

Organize the information

Reminder: Use the previously mentioned notebook, note cards, or bookmarks with information about each school, and write or print some or all of the aforementioned details in it so you can have the information when you need it, which becomes really important just before the interview (see this chapter for a template). Additionally, you may want to reproduce and print the included *note card* and *check-off sheet* for each school -- for quick reference. You may choose to make folders with printed pages from the schools' websites. You may want to type out information that can be combined with the website information or only use the following short note card format. It is up to you how to organize the school's information, but I would find a way to keep it organized and accessible. Murphy's Law may visit you just as the application deadline approaches. You may have exams, work, family commitments, and other time constraints that could make the process stressful. If your school information is neat and uncluttered, you will not feel as stressed as the deadlines approach. I recommend using the sample check-off sheets, for each school, and documenting your application progress as you complete each required step. Then place the respective, completed sheets in the front of each school's physical or e-folder you made. Be sure to keep all fax confirmations, emails, scans, and all postal certificates as well. Place this information in each school's respective folder, both as a hard-copy and by scanning it and storing it in a cloud-based manner such as *Drop Box* or *Google Drive*. By storing it all digitally, you can have the information you need at any time and in any place, where it may be suddenly needed. A school program director may email you one day, stating he/she does not have a vital piece of information. He/she may need the missing document(s) by the end of the day and if you have it neatly organized and accessible via an internet connection, or in a physical folder, you are prepared and can send it to him/her right away. This storage and organization could mean the difference between getting into school or not.

Example information on the "School Information Note Card" on the next page.

Example information on the "School Information Note Card"
Note: Format may be off due to size of your device or reader.

School Name:	website:
Location:	State:
Contact:	Phone: ( ) -
Email: @	Fax: ( ) -
App deadline date: / /	Start date: / /
Graduation date: / /	or estimate:
Unique classes needed to apply:	
School strengths/specialty:	
Tuition costs: $ /year, $ /semester, $ total	
Living expenses for area (high, low, equal):	
Scholarships?	
Positives (jobs, student's statements, family, reputation, etc., costs):	
Negatives/Barriers:	
Notes:	
Location info:	
Your personal rank of this school as a choice (circle one)	
This school is my: # 1 2 3 4 5 6 7 8 9 10	
Why:	

Example information on the "School Check off sheet"
Note: Format may be off due to size of your device or reader.

Therapy School Name:
Application completed and sent: Y / N
Date submitted: /   /   Deadline date: /   /
Receipt for Fed-ex/UPS/USPS: #
School contact person:
Contact info: @   (   )   -
Reference #1   Contact:
Completed: Y / N   Date submitted: /   /
Reference #2   Contact:
Completed: Y / N   Date submitted: /   /
Reference #3   Contact:
Completed: Y / N   Date submitted: /   /
Transcripts sent: School 1:   Date submitted: / /
Transcripts sent: School 2:   Date submitted: / /
Transcripts sent: School 3:   Date submitted: / /
Transcripts sent: School 4:   Date submitted: / /
GRE sent: Y / N   Date submitted:
Observation hours -- forms completed and sent: /   /
Site: Y / N   Date submitted: /   /
Site: Y / N   Date submitted: /   /
Site: Y / N   Date submitted: /   /
Site: Y / N   Date submitted: /   /

Essay(s) completed: Y / N
Notes:

Ch. 3 Summary:

- Pick a degree you will still enjoy if you do not get into a professional therapy school.
- Know the schools that fit your abilities based on the school's requirements and location.
- Pick 5-10 schools you wish to apply to.
- Organize the information for each school so that you can access it physically and digitally.
- Interview the faculty and students to get to know them and to gain insight into the nuances of their schools.

Chapter 4

Physical Therapy Assistant

Becoming a physical therapy assistant or PTA is also an amazing choice for many aspiring health-care workers. The Bureau of Labor and Statistics states, "Physical therapist assistants (sometimes called PTAs) and physical therapist aides work under the direction and supervision of physical therapists. They help patients who are recovering from injuries and illnesses regain movement and manage pain." The Bureau also states, that. . . "Most states require physical therapist assistants to have an associate's degree from an accredited physical therapist assistant program. Physical therapist aides generally have a high school diploma and receive on-the-job training" The median income for a PTA was around $54,000 of the estimated 76,910 PTA's employed as of May 2014. The expected growth rate follows the positive growth rate of P.T.'s and O.T.'s. PTAs provide many of the same physical therapy techniques based on the physical therapist's plan of care. The PTA will follow that plan of care (POC) and provided treatment based on the PT's determination of the appropriate intervention(s). Some common interventions used are: activities of daily living training, therapeutic exercise, manual techniques, gait training, prosthetic training, deep soft tissue massage, and modalities such as heat, ice, electrotherapy and ultrasound.

Schools: There are ~ 311 accredited PTA programs in the continental USA with one in Hawaii and four in Puerto Rico totaling

316. See: The CAPTE website for details at http://www.capteonline.org/Programs/

Curriculum per the APTA:

> The length of a PTA program is typically 2 years (5 semesters) consisting of general education course, physical therapy courses, and clinical education. Primary physical therapy content areas in the curriculum may include, but are not limited to, anatomy & physiology, exercise physiology, biomechanics, kinesiology, neuroscience, clinical pathology, behavioral sciences, communication, and ethics/values. Approximately seventy-five percent (75%) of the PTA curriculum comprises classroom (didactic) and lab study and the remaining 25 percent (25%) is dedicated to clinical education. PTA students spend on average 16 weeks in full-time clinical education experiences.

Most schools will require a 3.0 ("B" average) in the prerequisite courses such as: anatomy and physiology, math, psychology, humanities, but these vary widely and you **must** contact the program director to find which classes are needed and what grades are required. Note: Some schools require at least a "C" in these courses.

Per the APTA the licensure/certification is as follows: "After graduation from an accredited physical therapy education program* candidates must pass a state-administered national exam to obtain licensure or certification required in most states. Other requirements vary from state to state according to physical therapy practice acts or state regulations governing physical therapy. Visit the Federation of State Boards of Physical Therapy (FSBPT) Web site for more information about PTA licensure/certification requirements."

Certified Occupational Therapy Assistant (COTA)

As described by the US Bureau for Labor Statistics, occupational therapy assistants and aides help patients develop, recover, and improve the skills needed for daily living and working. Occupational therapy assistants are directly involved in providing therapy to patients, while occupational therapy aides typically perform support activities. Both assistants and aides work under the direction of occupational therapists.

The Bureau also states: "Occupational therapy assistants need an associate's degree from an accredited occupational therapy assistant program. In most states, occupational therapy assistants must be licensed."

In May of 2012 the Bureau reports a median income of $53,240 for a COTA and employment of occupational therapy assistants and aides is projected to grow 41 percent from 2012 to 2022.

As of March 2013, there were 162 occupational therapy assistant programs accredited by the Accreditation Council for Occupational Therapy Education. www.aota.org/education-careers.

The prerequisites are very similar to the PTA programs, but these vary widely and you **must** contact the program director to find which classes are needed and what grades are required.

Chapter 5

Academics

After reading the previous chapters, you now know how important grades are. You have likely heard that all you need is the diploma and that it alone will open doors for you. This is not entirely true, but many employers will base hiring only on the interview and your résumé. Most employers, however, will screen applicants based on grades, and accomplishments, but will consider other factors such as a student who worked his or her way through college, or was in athletics while in college. Many employers will check references, run background checks, and drug screens. You are applying to graduate school and need to show you are a competitive and serious candidate, just like an applicant to a professional job. Even if you do work while in college, you still need to keep greater than a 3.5 GPA, if possible. Your grades are looked at first and used to decide whether or not you make the cut. Passing a state or national board exam is required for a therapist to practice. This is one more reason to make great grades in P.T. or O.T. school as a solid foundation for the board exam. Note: If you have a felonious past, you will not be allowed to take most state board exams.

Grades do matter

I cannot emphasize enough how hard you need to work during your high school and college years to even get the opportunity to interview for a physical or occupational therapy school. How do you to make the grades needed? Pick a major you are interested in and do not overload your schedule by taking too many hours. If you choose a non-science major, you will need to take more science electives to meet the professional school's requirements. In all things, there is a balance. Find it. It is easier to make great grades if you only take two or three classes per semester, but it will take too long. The opposite is true if you try to take over twenty hours your first semester and make only average grades. Find the balance between the extremes.

What not to do

Missing class: College students are usually on tight budgets and we all want to get what we pay for, but college classes may be the only instance where you pay for something and choose not to take advantage of it. On average, the public tuition and fees for a four-year university are around $9,000 per year based on a 15-hour semester. That comes out to $600 per class hour or $1800 for a three-hour course. Over a 15-week semester, you would meet 30-45 times at $60 or $40 per class, respectfully. Even if *you* are not paying for it, someone is. You should respect that and get the information that is due to you. If you miss one day (three classes), you just lost up to $180; miss one week and you paid around $600 for nothing and received no instruction. You will most likely ruin a reference from that professor as well. Lack of interaction with the teaching assistants and professors is also a negative, because they will not know you. Not taking the class seriously or believing, "I will never use this information," is a bad idea. You need to put all you can into your studies as if your career depends upon it.

Start as early as possible

As far as grades go, start your freshman year and do all you can to ensure that you have the highest grades you can honestly get. If you are reading this while still in high school, then take more advanced math and science classes to better prepare yourself for the more rigorous college courses. You will have to work hard all through college to do this. That means when you are studying for tomorrow's physics test and your friends ask you to meet them at the river or at a party, you should decline and think about the P.T. or O.T. school applicant who will get your spot because he or she had a higher GPA. You can always go out sometime after your exam. I would also recommend that you go to preparation courses for the GRE to increase your odds in the application process. This is a career that will pay you 65 to 90+ thousand dollars per year; you should put into it what you will get back. After twenty years in this career, you will have likely earned one to two million dollars. This is just the monetary end of this field. The spiritual rewards and happiness in a career, where you change people's lives for the better, is truly priceless. I suggest putting serious study time for your five to seven years of school so that you can enjoy the fruits of that labor, for many years after graduating. It is more than worth it.

Grades take a time investment

Making high grades takes an immense amount of self-discipline. I learned early on that if I read my history class chapters four times, then I aced the exam. I read the notes or textbook the first time and highlighted in yellow, the next time I re-read and noticed more than a few things I missed and I highlighted those in orange. Then, on the third read, it became more of a slow skim with a few things that had not stuck - now using green to highlight. Lastly, I was able to use a fast skim and highlighted a few forgotten sentences or words in pink. On the morning of the exam, I did a quick skim of mostly the pink highlights. The information was now more engrained. I recommend this layering type of learning because the material is not crammed in and then quickly forgotten. For example, I recommend studying Monday's notes on Monday, then Monday's <u>and</u> Wednesday's notes on Wednesday and so on. By the time the first exam comes, you have re-skimmed the information so many times that you do not have to stress or cram to ace it. Think of how smoothly a comprehensive final exam will go if you do not have to cram the four previous months of notes and readings back in your memory. My philosophy about making good grades started while taking EMT classes in my early college career. As an EMT, you literally hold life in your hands. What if you retain only a portion of what you are taught? Which EMT or paramedic would you want responsible for saving your life: the one who crammed or the one who really studied it, over and over? By layering the information, the material will be permeated and thus, you will remember it much longer.

Ch. 5 Summary

- Pick a degree plan and courses you enjoy.
- Balance your work and school hours.
- Study daily, layering the information.
- Practice delayed gratification.
    - Work hard for 5-7 years to enjoy a career for a lifetime.
- Finally, graduate with a 3.5 or greater GPA.

Chapter 6

Volunteering and Employment

The volunteers and interns we note as hire-worthy are the ones who quickly show their outgoing, but appropriate personalities. These individuals find a balance and are very confident, but not arrogant. Too quiet and the therapists never get to know you. Too arrogant and they quickly do not trust you, because you become a potential hazard by trying to do things you are not trained in. Over confidence will also irritate veteran technicians who clearly know more about their clinical environment than the new, overbearing volunteer. As a new volunteer or intern, do not be mousey and flinch when talked to, nor should you try to speak authoritatively about topics that you know very little about.

Successful or not?

The most successful applicants prior, during, and after becoming physical or occupational therapists are those individuals who give of themselves first. The unsuccessful individuals look for what they can extract from their environment. For example, they come in the therapy facility just to fulfill hourly requirements and then go home. This career will give back so much to you if you genuinely put others first. These genuine individuals are cheerful, motivated, and excited to help all those they serve. My advice is that these potential future therapists should quickly get used to putting the patients first, then the company, and lastly the employees and physicians. The individuals that do this honestly, stand out quickly. They are the ones who willingly stay late, eagerly work hard, and soak up every bit of information possible. They have done their homework, are aware of the field and the clinical setting; they are taking all the steps necessary to achieve their goals. These aspiring individuals have the foresight to make great grades because they understand the delayed gratification that they can expect. I notice the volunteer or interns who work hard to be a vital cog in the *machine* of the clinic operation; they serve the patient's and clinic's needs with true and undying enthusiasm. The opposite of this is demonstrated in those who are only volunteering to get their hours documented, and then leave at or before closing. This uninspiring group may fiddle with their phones, talk to each other about current events or their classes, stare into space, and walk around the clinic doing nothing. They choose this behavior instead of learning in the clinic. The successful ones communicate with the staff and the patients effectively, both verbally and non-verbally. If they have to miss a shift or leave early, they will have truly convinced me why. Notice I said convinced, since some will tell you weekly excuses as to why they have to leave early or why they cannot come in. The good ones stay and help without saying a word and have to be reminded of things like, "don't you have to be at your other job or class now?" The unsuccessful ones will just leave early and hope no one notices.

However, there is the classic category of volunteers or interns who operate at a unique extreme. They are the ones who can be so overt and pushy that they irritate the therapists, employees, and patients. I have seen some new volunteers who act as if they have known the therapist and the patients for years. They behave too familiar too quickly, which makes everyone around them uncomfortable. This behavior tends to be distracting and an interruption – don't do this. Again, there must be a balance. This is a misunderstood pearl among the many suggestions that you will be told in the pursuit of this field. It is universal and should be applied in all things – balance.

> Note: Keeping things in balance can make or break you in most situations. As a new volunteer or intern, work your way in slowly with the patients and staff, impressing them with your dedication.

Human instincts are a vital guide that we sometimes ignore. An example in the animal world is when a dog approaches another dog's turf. A smart dog will assess the other dogs and find his/her place in the pack. Once accepted into the area, the new dog has to observe and remain submissive until his or her time comes to exert a more prominent role, if possible. This rule is true with interactions with people while at work, school, and at social events.

We have all known the new person who comes into a group, whether at work or socially, who is too overt and acts as if he/she is already very well known. The other extreme is the new person who never opens up at all and remains on the outside of the established group, literally and emotionally. You must find your interactive balance and vary it daily, keenly observing the established group's stress level or frivolity. When the clinical staff is busy and stressed, keep your head down and help them as efficiently as possible. If you do not know how to help, try to observe what the staff is doing and assess whether you can directly help or not. Sometimes just keeping things clean and organized is very helpful for the technicians and therapists. In my practice setting, the minutes add up. If you save my technicians one to two minutes every hour, then by the end of the day we all may be able to leave on time and be with our friends or families. We quickly notice the volunteers or interns that "chat-it-up" with others about their day, their classes, and their hobbies, thereby distracting others from learning or helping. It is frustrating to need assistance from an employee who is drawn into a conversation about non-work related topics and even work topics, if the timing is poor. The therapists do not expect or want you to only do menial labor; we want to see your interests in the field of therapy. You should demonstrate your natural curiosity by observing treatment and evaluations. Please ask the therapists if you can observe and ask the patient as well. Do not sheepishly stand a few feet away without introducing yourself or indicating what your role is in the facility. Example, "Hello, my name is Heidi, and I am an observer. Do you mind if I sit in and watch the evaluation?" Settings vary and some clinicians allow the volunteers to do multiple tasks, while others only allow observation. Find your place, regardless of the setting, and help if you are allowed. If the aides do much of the prep work, then help them. If the therapist is working alone, quickly learn how to make that clinician more efficient. Take the initiative and learn where everything (towels, sheets, instruments, modalities) is located so you are able to get it to the therapist thus allowing him or her to work more efficiently. Let the therapist and staff know what you have learned, and offer to help.

Hint: Get the therapist to write your recommendation close to the end of your time with him/her, or very soon after you have moved on. Remind the therapist that he/she knows you best at this time and it will be easier for him/her to write about you if this is done sooner rather than later. If he/she is not willing or able to write your letter this soon, ask if he/she would consider jotting down and keeping a few notes about you. I suggest that you write your own brief self-summary that shows your grades, the steps you have taken demonstrating your dedication, and lastly, any contributions you have made to that clinical setting. This is like a brief résumé that is specific to your time with the therapist(s) and will help you obtain a stellar recommendation letter. Early in your volunteering or even before you volunteer, intern, or work at a clinic, look up the recommendation forms at the schools in which you will apply. These forms have multiple categories and scoring for things like appearance, critical thinking, communication, and more. Print the forms and study what you will be rated on. Try to hone your skills and look for genuine clinical opportunities to excel in these specific criteria. Be sure to do this well in advance of when the therapists will actually rate/grade you.

Hint: If you always give cheerfully, you will get glowing reviews. As President Kennedy once said, "Ask not what your country can do for you — ask what you can do for your country." Apply this principle to the clinics, hospitals, patients, and therapists you interact with, and you will impress all you encounter. The therapist will notice you over those volunteers or interns who are unable to genuinely do this. As one who has written hundreds of these letters, I can tell you that this helps your recommendation forms/letters in every way.

Ch. 6 Summary:

- Be a cheerful and honest giver of your time, enthusiasm, and energy. Learn your place and stand out as that someone everyone can rely on to make the facility run better.
- Do not distract the therapists, staff, or patients.
- Become the go-to person by being eager and willing to help 100% of the time and do the tasks as effectively and independently as possible.
  - We will easily remember you, if you become this person!
  - Be proactive regarding the recommendation letter you will need to get into therapy school.

Chapter 7

Civic Duties

These duties would entail the moral, legal, and physical accountability of everyone to leave our communities in a better condition than we found them. To achieve this, we as members of society must do our part to help. This can, and likely should be, in the form of the person's passion. Some of us love animals and can help at shelters; others like construction and help with projects like Habitat for Humanity. We all should be good stewards of the earth, our country, our state, our city, and our local communities. Doing this is not just for the hours to make you look good; it is about truly making a difference. If you have not yet volunteered, then you have not experienced the *good feeling* because you have made a difference and helped better someone or something. You could go to **volunteermatch.org** and find the type of local opportunity that will not just benefit those you help, but will change you, at least a little, for the better. If you really want to stand out on interviews, being a volunteer is good, but being a leader with a title is better. Examples: Treasurer of the Pre-P.T. club at school or Head Coordinator of PAWS local chapter. Be a leader in whatever you do, it makes a difference. You have to stand out against a very competitive crowd that the interviewers will be reviewing on interview day. These fellow applicants have also done civic duties; some even started his/her duties back in high school. Start early, in middle or high-school where you can learn quickly the traits of a good steward of your community and consequently, benefit your soul. Starting early in this process also builds your resume which helps you in all future aspects of school and job applications.

Chapter 8

Recommendation Letters

You will need multiple recommendation letters from therapists and professors. Check with the schools to see if they require at least one or two letters from practicing therapists. I have interviewed an applicant that had two letters from one therapist, which failed to meet the school's instruction, thus precluding her from admittance. Some schools accept letters from others who have a lofty position in their field such as physicians or politicians. These individuals should know you very well. If they don't, your letter will feel flat (even though the author is well known) and it will be obvious to the reader that the writer does *not* know *you* very well. This type of letter is mostly worthless to you and to the school reviewer reading it.

As discussed earlier, you should ask the person writing your letter to jot down a few notes about you if he/she plans to write your letter at a future time. Remember to give him/her a summary of your accomplishments and contributions you made, both at the writer's class, clinic, or department. You should also include things that you have accomplished outside of the professor's or clinician's realm that reveal you in a positive light. It is extremely important that you give 100% every time you are working with that individual and your community. You need to show him or her your best side, but more importantly you need to submerse yourself into being an honest helper and hard worker so it becomes who you are. We see through the thin veil of a volunteer or intern who is just pretending to be helpful and nice. It is painfully obvious and your peers will pick up on it too. Do not discount the benefits of helping your fellow volunteers, interns, and the technicians as well. We may ask your peers and our technicians what they think of the new volunteer or intern. If a professor is going to write a recommendation, then you should have a good rapport with him/her and you should have shown the writer your work ethic by your grades, your office visits, and by previously seeking his or her advice.

> Note: Do not ask questions in class that you and everyone obviously know the answer to, just to "show" the professor you are there. Do ask occasional, "real," unique, and helpful questions. You should be known by name or deed for the letter of recommendation to have any substance.

What not to do: Come to the clinician or professor one or two days before the deadline for school admission, wanting a recommendation letter. This is a bad idea because it puts the therapist or professor in a time crunch and will likely irritate them. Therefore, your letter is not as good as it could be if it gets written at all. Even worse are the candidates who do not know the therapist or professor very well, and even though the candidate is made aware of this fact by the author, the applicant seeking the letter still wants a written recommendation. Some of these candidates have been told by the therapist or professor that they cannot write a favorable letter, but the applicant still insists it be written for him/her because without a letter, he/she will not be able to apply to school. I highly advise applicants not to procrastinate or ask for a letter from a therapist or professor who does not know the applicant very well. Your letter will be all but worthless to the reviewers at the professional school. Without a good letter of recommendation, the applicant should count on a rejection email in their future.

As mentioned earlier, it can be very helpful to write your own brief self-summary that shows your grades, the steps you have taken that demonstrate your dedication, and lastly, any contributions you have made to that clinical setting. This brief résumé, that is specific to your time with the therapist(s), will help you obtain a stellar recommendation letter. As also stated previously, it is very proactive and will make you stand out compared to others. It is very important for you to look up the recommendation forms from the schools in which you will apply, and use these forms as a guide for your behavior and actions. Print the forms and study what you will be rated on. Remember, common locations that you will use to apply to many schools are **PTCAS** and **OTCAS**. The Physical Therapist Centralized Application Service (PTCAS) is a service of the American Physical Therapy Association (**APTA**), where you will find reference instructions for many schools. Some schools have PDF files you can download, print and give to the professor or the clinician to complete. You should let them know: 1) if they are to give the completed forms back to you in a sealed, signed envelope or 2) if they can just fax or email it directly to the institution. Remember: At the centralized application site you can get the deadlines, prerequisites for each school and much more. Go to each school you are applying to and check prerequisites there as well.

A sample reference form from Texas State University P.T. program is located at:

1. http://www.health.txstate.edu/pt/admissions/applications.html

A sample from the UTHSCSA O.T. program is located at:

2. **http://shpwelcome.uthscsa.edu/ot/ot_ac.asp**

Please note, websites change frequently and these and all links may cease to function in the future.

You <u>must</u> stay in touch with each of the therapists you worked under, and each of the faculty members you will want a reference letter from. If you don't stay in touch, these professionals may forget important details about you. I have had volunteers whom I had not seen or heard from in three years contact me for reference letters. Three years is a long time to try to remember specifics about a person who may have only been in the clinic for 60 or 70 hours. Do not do this. Stop by and say hello, reintroduce yourself periodically, and genuinely ask how these potential reference writers are doing. At our clinic, I take a picture of each new volunteer and keep them in folders, and name the folder "current" and after they finish their rotation with us, they are placed in distinct folders by the year in which they volunteered or interned. You may find a way to have your picture available for the author, so he/she can remember you easier. I would include it in the résumé you developed for him/her and explain that the picture may help the writer recall details about you in the future. You may know of a hobby or passion the writer has. Genuinely inquire how that is going. Be honest and let him or her know that eventually you would really appreciate a *great* reference letter in the future. Please be aware that this takes time for the writers and you should respect and acknowledge this with much gratitude. Do not come in during a busy time and say something like, "I need this today" or "I need you to do this" and just set it down on their desk. I have had this done to me plenty of times and it is one of the worst things you can do as an aspiring therapist, because it shows your immaturity and lack of respect of the therapist's time.

Hint: Ask them if they honestly know you well enough to write a *very good* letter for you. Remember: when you bring the reference material to the therapist or faculty member, please have pre-addressed, stamped envelopes, and fill out all the form fields where applicable. You can fill in the therapist's name or the professor's name with the appropriate title, his/her address, email, how long you have known them, and anything else you can write or type so the writer of your recommendation does not need to. This extra effort will show your respect for their time. Give them all the forms, if applying to multiple schools, in a folder with detailed instructions for each school. You want to make this as easy for them as possible. I recommend an included check-off sheet so he or she can easily see and check off each step required/completed. Also have a pre-addressed, stamped envelope for each school. Be sure to put your contact information in it so they can contact you if questions arise. The check-off sheet you made for them should include all the materials needed for each school, such as hours documented and of course, the reference form. It should include where, how, and when the materials should be sent, and the deadline dates for each school. Let the writer know when you will check back with him or her to check on the status. I recommend checking back with the writers one to two weeks before the application due date. Some professors and therapists are very busy and need to be pushed a little to ensure your forms get completed on time. I know an applicant that had to make multiple calls to the therapist and meet the therapist at his workplace to get the completed form the same day it was due.

See the following example of a recommendation letter request.

SAMPLE LETTER TO PUT ON LEFT SIDE OF FOLDER

1-17-2015

Regarding Recommendation Letter(s) for: "Your name"

Dear Mr./Mrs./Dr. "Smith,"

Thank you in advance! It was a pleasure speaking with you (last week, yesterday or whenever) about my recommendation letters. I truly appreciate your time and willingness to write these letters for [P.T./O.T.] school. I know how busy you are, and it means a great deal that you would take the time to do write these for me. Since two of the schools I am applying for request recommendations online, please be aware and look for emails from [university(s) name].

I have enclosed a folder with all the form(s), my resume, and the activities I performed at your clinic. I feel these documents will be very helpful for you regarding my recommendations.

I have enclosed my rec. letter forms from Texas State.

You can check off in the "___" (space) when you complete each of these forms, if that helps.

- For UNT: ___complete on-line assessment and submit electronically by 10-1-13.
- For Texas State: ___ complete the enclosed form, sign and date, seal in the enclosed, stamped envelope, and sign across the seal. Keep that one, and I will pick it up on Wednesday the 15th at lunch, if that works for you.
- For Duke: ___ complete on-line assessment and submit electronically by 10-14-13.

Thank you again, and if you have any questions, please call or text me at:

Cell: 830-777-####

My email is: **PTwannabe@yehaw.pt**

John Smith

John Smith

P.S. I will email you Sept. 29th to check on UNT, and on the 10th to check on Duke, and lastly I will see you on the 15th for Texas State.

END OF SAMPLE LETTER

Ch. 8 Summary:

- Be known to the therapist or professor.
- Write a summary about yourself and give it to them for reference.
- Ask them to make notes about you.
- Give 100% all the time.
- Do not procrastinate.
- Know the school's reference form's criteria <u>before</u> observing and work on doing them well so you can get a stellar recommendation.
- Make it easy for the reference form writer by leaving him/her plenty of time to complete it and filling in as much information on the forms as you can.
  - Organize it well so it is easy for the writer to complete each step.

Chapter 9

The Interview

Now that you have prepared well academically, met all the application requirements, and met all deadlines, you may then be asked to interview. You will need an outstanding interview to be accepted. This is much more difficult than you can imagine. I have sat in on hundreds of interviews and witnessed what it takes to stand out and what makes the interview just mediocre. I have also personally witnessed and have learned about interviews in which the school faculty had no choice but to decline the applicant due to the candidate's undesirable behavior. These applicants were either blatantly crude to someone in the department, dressed inappropriately, or had poor attitudes. Other applicants had more subtle issues, but were still unsuccessful, because they responded neutrally, bland, and were lacking confidence. The other reason applicants do poorly, during interviews, is due to a general lack of knowledge about the field of physical or occupational therapy.

> Note: In my opinion, this is the hardest part of the entire process because it all boils down to a 20-30 minute period that defines your future as a P.T. or O.T.

You really need to do your homework as mentioned previously. Homework equals knowing the field of P.T. or O.T. extremely well so that you can speak about it very easily and naturally. It means you know all about the university, the professors, and all steps needed to be successful. It also means knowing yourself and the role you are hoping to fill as a therapist.

I just spoke with a great applicant last night during my entire 30 minute commute home. She told me she has an interview tomorrow morning and wanted to talk about interview tips. She had studied the field very well, but when I asked her to tell me why she chose that out of state program, she stammered some. I told her, "You have to be able to paint a verbal picture of why you chose that school, why it is a good choice, and what you will offer them." I further explained that the interviewers need to see the steps you have taken to improve your standing, since this was not her first time to apply, and that she needs to convey her future role in the field and at that school. I told her that the interviewers need to see that you have taken all the steps necessary, and have worked on improving any deficits. Some improvements may be: re-taking classes, expanding your volunteer setting variety, understanding the practice of P.T. or O.T. and studying the respective political arena(s). Essentially, they want to see that you have done all your homework, are improving yourself on deficits, and have a solid plan to succeed.

Necessary attributes

In addition, you have to be comfortable in your own skin. This means you have to know yourself and exhibit confidence. Without this, you do not come across naturally. The best applicants are very open, honest, and make solid eye contact. Great applicants "sparkle." You must be comfortable in what you know about the program, yourself, and the profession. This means you study and know it cold, even under the pressure of the interview. To *sparkle*, you have to be happy, excited, and truly passionate about this current opportunity to become a therapist. You will have to show this while you engage the interviewers sitting across from you. I suggest repeated mock interviews with friends, family, or perhaps at your school library where it can be video-recorded. Review the recordings yourself and get feedback from therapists, faculty, leaders in their fields, and your family. Hint: Download and print as many sample questions you can find and practice answering them. Your answers should be polished, but honest and come from you, not what you would say to try to impress the faculty.

> Note: Practice making almost constant eye contact with everyone in the room if either you or they are speaking.

We must face the fact that some people are just more charismatic than others due to their upbringing, genetics, or both. Being naturally charismatic is definitely a plus. You can work on this by practicing genuine concern for others and expressing it verbally and with your actions. For example, try practicing being engaged, listening, knowing your place, being helpful, working hard to serve, and joking about yourself. If you apply these principles, then at the interview you will be able to relax and not have to try so hard.

On-site behavior on interview day

Once you arrive at the school, consider every personal interaction as a mini interview – even if you think these people have nothing to do with your actual one-on-one interview. I have seen examples where the applicants were very boastful and cocky or just simply treated others badly. Two examples come to mind. The first was an applicant who did not consider that the faculty would soon find out about this poor behavior. The second example was an applicant that showed inappropriate public affection. Regarding behaviors, you should never be insincere; you need to transform your attitude now, and always show your best behavior. To be viewed in a positive light on interview day, you need to be noticed. My recommendation to applicants who are trying to get noticed is to work on fostering and developing a natural, happy, honest, respectful, and giving personality. You are the only one who can choose your attitude about life. Why not choose happiness and honesty? These traits are crucial for this career. The most content individuals are those who give of themselves. This field requires a happy demeanor and a giving spirit which the interviewers will notice quite quickly.

Stepping behind the door

Once you enter the interview room, you need to stand until asked to sit, greet interviewer(s) with solid eye contact, a smile, and give a firm handshake. Be prepared to talk with the interviewers about why you chose P.T. or O.T in the first place, and why you want to go to their school. Also consider what makes *you* a good fit for their program. Consider events or an event that swayed you into this career path. Consider how you work with others, how you have made a difference in someone's life, or a patient encounter that transformed you in some way. Consider how you handle stress and what your most and least favorite classes were. Think about the aforementioned questions and what you would say. You will likely be asked something you were not prepared to answer, like "What makes you stand out against the other applicants?" Be humble, (but not self-demeaning) since you are competing against equally qualified individuals. However, you have to be known as one with confidence and maturity. If you do not know the answer to one of the questions, you may even let them know that, and you may try to reason through it out loud so they can see how you think. The interviewers want to know if you are poised and prepared to answer their questions. Are you a problem solver and a critical thinker?

SELL YOUR POSITIVES! You are able to give the interviewers your point of view of why you make a great fit for the program. Be confident!

Common Questions

There are possibly hundreds of potential questions, but here are a few common ones:

1. Why did you choose physical therapy as a career over other health careers?
2. Why did you choose our school?
3. Describe a difficult situation you encountered, and how did you handle it?
4. Why should we choose you over the other applicants?
5. How is our school different than other schools you are applying to?
6. What are some important recent changes in the field of physical therapy?
7. What type of physical therapy setting do you plan to work in after graduation?
8. What would you do if you witnessed academic dishonesty in physical therapy school?

9. What are positives and negatives of direct access?

10. What are your strengths and weaknesses, and how have you addressed them?

11. How do you compare against others your age, regarding maturity?

12. What types of hobbies do you have?

13. What will you bring to our program that will make it better?

14. What will you do if you do not get in to a P.T. school this time?

Go to different school websites and download common P.T./O.T. school questions. Study them to give you an idea of what the questions could be like. Be specific with one to four sentence responses. You should not speak longer than one minute for most answers, but it is okay to speak longer if your "story" is interesting and the interviewers want to know how it ends. Try to be concise. You must be specific, using details, so you paint a picture with your words. If you play the guitar, don't say "my hobby is music." If you were an eagle scout on your 16th birthday, don't just tell the interviewers, "I was a boy scout." Be specific and tell your story so the interviewers are drawn in, and want to know more about you.

Note: BE POLITE! BE CONFIDENT! Answer them with: "Yes I do..., or No, I don't..., No sir, Yes ma'am," if in the South. Never say: "Uh-huh, Nope, Yeah, Nuh-uh" or anything else which would end in you performing push-ups as a punishment by a coach or drill sergeant.

SMILE and RELAX! Be grateful that you are there and show it. Most of all BE HONEST! Do not hesitate to accentuate your positives. Remember, the people sitting across from you used to be you! They had to get into school just like you are trying to do. They understand your position and nervousness. If you are the nervous-type in front of those in authority, then for that day, realize they likely had to go to the bathroom, just like you did. They stood and put their clothes on and drank coffee and ate breakfast, just like you did. They made it in, graduated, passed the board exam, and now teach and/or treat patients. You should imagine that you will get in and will know them later, so show genuine interest in these clinicians during the interview.

It is extremely important to show the interviewers that you understand the profession and current trends or changes such as direct access, the Medicare cap, Occupational Therapy Mental Health Act, Vision 2020, insurance trends and changes, doctoral graduates vs. master's graduates, and physician-owned clinics. Know the different roles that a P.T. or O.T. have as compared to the roles of P.T. or O.T. assistants. You should do your homework via the APTA and AOTA websites, *and* look at your own state's physical therapy association.

You need to dress appropriately for the interview, as if you are interviewing for a professional job. This equates to a suit and tie for men and business professional for women. Ask the chair, the professors, or current students what is expected for their school in particular. I would not wear any piercings and would minimize any visible tattoos. Be conservative with your cologne, perfumes, and jewelry. I am aware of applicants who had: Mohawks, bright crazy hair colors, deep cleavage, T-shirts, and even one who brought a spouse *into* the interview room. I would highly advise against what should be an obvious faux pas. The interview is the culmination of all your hard work – dress for it. Once sitting, speak with confidence. The interviewers need to be able to hear you clearly, see your eyes and your facial expressions. Study body language and apply it appropriately. Perform an internet search of: "body language at an interview."

Some obvious problematic examples are fidgeting, lack of eye contact, and talking nervously. This is a science with many more facets for you to consider and practice correctly. Review your recorded mock interviews to see if you sparkle, fidget, make eye contact, etc. Apply the positive body language aspects, while eradicating the negative ones.

The most important interview advice is to be honest and outgoing. Be grateful and show your gratitude for the opportunity you have. The people sitting across from you have to make the difficult decision of who gets past this interview and who does not. Ask them questions, but not too many, and give them a chance to ask you as many questions as they would like. This means you need to watch the time, without being obvious, and balance your talking so it is not too much or too little. Watch the interviewers to see if they start drifting during your answers, if so, you may be talking too much. If they are looking at you in a way that says, "Is there more?" then you may want to elaborate. Thank them graciously when you leave with a firm handshake and with something like, "Thank you so much for your time today, I really enjoyed this;" or "I hope to see you soon," said with a big smile. Some applicants have sent thank-you notes to the faculty the same day or very soon after the interview.

Ch. 9 Summary:

- This is one of the most important 20-30 minutes in the process.
- Be open, honest, and sparkle.
- Be comfortable in your own skin, you need to know: yourself, the field of therapy, the school, and the faculty.
- Consider every personal interaction at the school as a mini-interview.
- Show an honest, grateful attitude for the opportunity.
- Dress for the interview.
- Know body language and apply it appropriately.
- Be grateful for the interviewer's time.
- Don't talk too much or too little.
- Be sincere 100% of the time.

Chapter 10

Summary

Being a therapist is an amazing and life changing profession. It is well worth the preliminary investment of time, studies, volunteering, and research to achieve this endeavor. You need to do a few things first, before beginning this journey. You need to spend time observing in multiple therapy settings. This is your first step to determine if you like the career enough to pursue it. Ultimately, you want to love your career. You need to already possess or develop a giving, altruistic personality. You have to avoid distractions and study diligently prior to and during your P.T. or O.T. program. You will need to have at least a 3.5 grade-point average if possible. Make good impressions by giving 100% in all volunteering or civic duties, and be genuinely charismatic. Help the people writing your reference letters by giving them written information about you, your endeavors, and your experience at the reference's site. Study the schools, study the professors, and commit much to memory. I recommend organizing your information by: making note cards, folders, and by storing the web site data for each of the programs you are applying to. Organize your application process for quick reference. I did not cover essay letters because it is general information and can be addressed easily with other books and internet searches. I highly recommend you study and even print out three to five website pages that address essays and apply them when you write it. Write them well in advance because of the editing and re-editing that will be needed. Most schools will require one or two distinct essays or statements. Most are less than 500 words, since reviewers do not have the time to read hundreds of very long essays. The schools will usually ask one or two questions related to the field of therapy, you, or the school's program. You need to show your passion and try to be specific and unique here. Please write and re-write your essays with as many qualified editors as you can get to proofread for you. These essays are usually one to two pages which, like the interview, can make or break you. Lastly, stay in touch with each of the therapists you worked under and each of the faculty members you will want a reference letter from. Be charismatic and work on your interviewing skills. Practice giving and honing your work ethic.

Good luck, and I hope to see you practicing your dream one day.

Kirk Painter, PT, DPT, Cert. MDT

Special thanks to the many who have helped make this book better.

My wife Heidi; my Mom; Kelsey (my talented daughter); Jaishree; Sharon; Lori; Leslie; Sarah; and all the P.T.s and O.T.s listed in this book who were very helpful and made it more readable.

Made in the USA
Middletown, DE
19 June 2017